WORKBOOK FOR

CHANGE YOUR MIND

(A Guide to RJ Spina's Book)

Your Powerful Guide to Deprogramming your Subconscious Mind, Rewire the Brain and Balance your Energy

ALL RIGHTS RESERVED...

<u>ABOUT RJ SPINA</u>

There has never been a time when the world needs a leader and metaphysical teacher like RJ Spina more. He has cured himself, on the basis of his own true transcendence, of paralysis from the chest down, severe chronic sickness, and life-threatening disorders.

Many people's lives have been transformed and saved thanks to his teachings, knowledge, guidance, and revolutionary self-healing and self-realization technique.

He has devoted his life to the spiritual, emotional, and physical liberation and restoration of all people.

Put your preconceived notions aside and learn to bring about genuine healing. How to use energy healing to overcome suffering, find inner peace, and embrace the invincible Self is what RJ Spina shares after overcoming chest-down paralysis and chronic sickness.

To help you achieve your health and wellness objectives, including those linked to physical sickness, pain, depression, anxiety, addiction, and more, this book introduces a novel seven-step system for energetic attunement and neural rewiring.

In Supercharged Self-Healing, RJ and his clients introduce you to the Ascend the Frequencies Technique, a way to retrain your brain for better health.

Access higher realms of awareness and channel energy in a way that shuts off the program of illness with the help of this innovative book's guiding concepts and practices. This crucial manual uses guided imagery, meditation, and mantra practice to help you release your ego and live in the state of health and harmony that is your birthright.

When RJ was younger, he often found himself drawn to the mysterious spaces outside the range of human senses. He had a constant, profound feeling of knowledge that exceeded his rational capacity. As he struggled with 'regular' living at the age of twenty-four, he stumbled into a deep state of meditation.

That event was a watershed in RJ's development as a person. His own personal journey to freedom and self-awareness had begun with this direct experience and genuine comprehension.

**THIS ONE WEEK OUTLINE WAS
DEVELOPED TO HELP YOU.**

➢ The foremost thing
   is to find a
   person you can rely on to
   help you achieve your
   goals if you want to be
   successful.

➢ Be careful not
   to make any mistakes
   when filling out the vital
   forms displayed below.

➢ Consider each day's tip,
   task and prescription
   carefully.

**THINK ABOUT THEM
MEDITATIVELY.**

➢ **Everything you learned in the note should be written and meditated upon.**

Also, jot down your thoughts and feelings, as well as the obstacles you've come to terms with.

READ AND LISTEN TO
EVERYTHING
THAT IS BEING SAID
AND RECOMMENDED.

Without a doubt, adhere to
them.

IT WAS MADE TO BE
POSSIBLE.

Never doubt the fact that
you
can do it, and never give up
hope.

**YOU'RE ALL SET TO STEP
ON TO THE NEXT LEVEL!**

Ensure that you fill out the Form below in its entirety.

DATE IT ALL BEGINS

_____

_____

DATE OF FINAL CONCLUSION (Usually 7 D ays from the starting Date)

_____

Fill in the blanks with your name and email address:

_____

_____

FILL OUT YOUR AGE

_____

_____

It's not as difficult as you might
think, but don't take it for
granted and keep going.

Recommendations and
Tasks for the Day Don't End
That Day; Carry On and
Make Habits of Them.

DAY 1

INSIGHT

Understand today that you cannot be truly happy without money but you'd be happier than ever with money and without a job. As an adult, am sure nobody would be truly interested in catering for all your expenses.

WHAT YOU SHOULD IMBIBE TODAY

You need to add in more work once and for all to be getting some cash at least. Get a business model (passive income) that has the ability of generating sufficient revenue from nothing. I suggest listing a digital product to the market or an online service managed by others.

DON'T FORGET...

True happiness and freedom cannot
be attained without money, that'd be
self-deceit.

MEDITATE

_____

_____

_____

_____

_____

_____

_____

_____

_____

_____

_____

_____

_____

_____

_____

_____

_____

_____

_____

_____

_____

_____

_____

_____

_____

_____

_____

_____

_____

The prior step to this is getting 'automatic' money.

DAY 2

INSIGHT

Liberty and happiness does not come from idleness. Being busy during the day with hobbies, adventures, things and people you love is the way to this.

WHAT YOU SHOULD IMBIBE TODAY...

Find out those things you love doing that are good for you. Have a weekly plan of your hobbies, travels, adventures and hanging out with friends.

DON'T FORGET...

No idle and sane person can truly claim to be happy. We are human; we were made to be adventurous.

MEDITATE

_____
_____
_____
_____
_____
_____
_____
_____
_____
_____
_____
_____
_____
_____

_____

_____

_____

_____

_____

_____

_____

_____

_____

_____

_____

_____

The idle mind is indeed devil's workshop.

DAY 3

INSIGHT

Understand today that health is wealth, health is everything. A sick person can neither have happiness nor liberty.

WHAT YOU SHOULD IMBIBE TODAY

Put a stop to unhealthy lifestyle and practices. Stop drugs, smoking, alcohol and unhealthy diet. Stop all forms of unhealthy and unfavorable behaviors.

DON'T FORGET...

Don't ever jeopardize or compromise health for fun, you'd regret it terribly.

MEDITATE...

_____

_____

_____

_____

_____

_____

_____

_____

_____

_____

_____

_____

_____

_____

_____

_____

_____
_____
_____
_____
_____
_____
_____
_____
_____
_____
_____

Good health is your biggest asset.
_____

DAY 4

INSIGHT

Exercises and good night rest have been proven to put more light to your entire life. This lifestyle strengthens your cells and improves your happiness and freedom,

WHAT YOU SHOULD IMBIBE TODAY

Go to bed early, rise early and exercise your body every morning. This habit alone would add to your length of days and strength at old age.

DON'T FORGET...

Even if you don't have much
resources for a good life, practicing
good night rest and morning exercises
would help you stay good.

MEDITATE

_____

_____

_____

_____

_____

_____

_____

_____

_____

_____

_____

_____

_____

_____

_____

_____

_____

_____

_____

_____

_____

_____

_____

_____

_____

_____

_____

**Exercising and having a good
night rest isn't costly.**

DAY 5

INSIGHT

Overburdening yourself with life troubles (Both yours and those of others) is one of the best ways of living a miserable life..

WHAT YOU SHOULD IMBIBE TODAY...

Do the things you can do and leave the rest. You don't have to carry all burdens, they'd kill you sooner.

<u>DON'T FORGET</u>

If you die today, the world will still
forget you and move on despite how
important you might think you are.
Those problems would still be solved
one way or the other.

MEDITATE

_____

_____

_____

_____

_____

_____

_____

_____

_____

_____

_____

_____

_____

_____

_____

_____

_____

_____

_____

_____

_____

_____

_____

_____

_____

_____

Stop giving a f*ck.

DAY 6

INSIGHT

Your diet lifestyle has a very important role to play in your life and personal well-being. You should never forget this fact.

WHAT YOU SHOULD IMBIBE TODAY

Put an end to all forms of unhealthy diet today. Don't eat out of impulse. Get a healthy food plan and stick to eat.

DON'T FORGET

Bad feeding has negative impact on your health and well-being. End the consumption of bad food at all cost.

MEDITATE

_____

_____

_____

_____

_____

_____

_____

_____

_____

_____

_____

_____

_____

_____

_____

_____

_____

_____

_____

_____

_____

_____

_____

_____

_____

**Rather go hungry than eat
unhealthy dishes.**

DAY 7

INSIGHT

The place where you live or spend ample time has been proven to have great impact on your mood, health and general well-being. It is advisable to try as much as possible to live in comfortable, less toxic and neat places.

WHAT YOU SHOULD IMBIBE TODAY

If the place you live tarnishes your self-worth, emotions, and mood or saps your energy, leave there immediately. If it isn't neat and organized, put in the work now.

DON'T FORGET

Be neat at all times because
cleanliness is next to Godliness!!!

MEDITATE

_____

_____

_____

_____

_____

_____

_____

_____

_____

_____

_____

_____

_____

_____

_____

_____

_____

_____

_____

_____

_____

_____

_____

_____

_____

_____

_____

_____

The place you live tells a lot about you!

YOU'VE FINISHED WITHTHIS ONE WEEK GUIDE. KEEP UP WITH IT.

POSITIVE RESULT COMES WITH IT.

Show Love to people by giving them copies of this.

_____

_____

_____

_____

_____

_____

_____

_____

_____

_____

_____

_____

_____

_____

_____

_____

BYE!

Each time you're deviating, return to this!

Made in United States
Troutdale, OR
07/28/2024

21600767R00030